THE ABC'S
of
HOPE & HEALING

by Mariah Clark Skewes

A book for daily reflections.

A book of prompts for journal entries.

A book of discussion starters for groups.

A book to be gifted to oneself or others.

A book to supplement, not supplant, counseling or therapy.

A book to offer hope and healing.

Dedicated to Anna & Mark.

We made it.

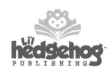

Li'l hedgehog
PUBLISHING

A

Acknowledge
Acknowledge your hurt.
Acknowledge your Anxiety or your Anger.
Acknowledge the Absence, Abuse, Alcoholism,
chaos, incarceration, chemical use,
depression, mental illness or other shortcomings
of those who hurt you.
Acknowledge that they were imperfect people,
dealing with their own unresolved issues.
Acknowledgement
is the first step toward healing.

B

Believe
Believe that you can become the person
you want to Be.
Believe that you can heal and move on.
Believe that you can
Break the cycle.
Believe that you can create a positive future for yourself.
Believe that life
is worth living.

C

Confide

Confide in a person you can trust.

A Counselor, therapist, or friend,

the parent of a friend,

a neighbor, or a relative.

A person in your Church, temple or mosque.

Find a Confidante with whom you can be honest,

who is worthy of your trust.

And rely on their

Counsel.

D

Decide

Decide that you are going to move forward
to change your circumstances.
Decide that you will work hard –
and it will be hard work.
Decide to surround yourself with positive people who
can help you on your journey.
Decide & Distance yourself from those
who would pull you back.

E

Embark

Embark on a journey of seeking

guidance and help.

Embark on a journey of recovery and hope.

Embark on a journey to

End the cycle of confusion, addiction, or hopelessness.

Embark on a journey to

Establish a new and more positive

you.

F

Focus

Focus on the Future.

The past is just that - the past.

It cannot be changed.

But the Future is yours to create.

Past Failures do not have to be repeated or define you.

You can learn from them.

Forgive where you can.

Let the Failures go and move on

to a brighter and more positive Future.

G

Go for it!

Set Goals and work toward them.

Start small - fulfilling today's responsibilities -

Get up, Go to school/work/appointments;

Get chores done.

Experience a bit of daily success and then expand.

Good Grades; Graduation; career training; college; job;

your own housing.

And Give Gratitude for your successes along the way.

H

Hope

Have Hope!

Things WILL get better.

Life won't always seem so gray and sad

as it has in the past or as it may right now.

Have Hope for a better tomorrow.

Have Hope for positivity, for calm,

for serenity.

Have Hope for Happiness and joy.

I

use 'I statements'

"I am working on ..."   "I am hurt when you ..."

"I have decided I am going to ..."

I statements allow you to take responsibility for yourself -

without blaming others.

Try "I've decided it's best for me not to

see you anymore," rather than -

"You're responsible for my unhappiness."

No judgment, just taking responsibility

for what's best

for YOU.

J

Journal

Journaling allows you to think, to reflect.

Jot down your losses, fears, anger, and frustrations,

your failures, insecurities, dreams, and triumphs.

Keep your Journal safe -

and if you're concerned about privacy,

destroy each page after you write it.

It is the writing that releases you.

Just give it a try.

K

Keep going

There are days when just getting out of bed
seems impossible. But you can do it!
Get up, get dressed, look at the day's responsibilities,
and get them done - One by one.
Showing up is the Key - it's half the battle.
And it's easier once you start.
Get some momentum going!
Keep going!

L

Let it be
Leave the negative relationships behind.
Don't engage.
Don't take responsibility for others or their actions
or their choices - just for yourself.
You can't change others.
Let go of the anger, the fears, the frustrations.
Leave the negative thoughts of blame behind.
Let time pass and Let healing begin.

M

Mentor

Find a Mentor -
a person who Models what you hope to be.
Confident, successful, assured, responsible,
kind, respectful.
Model yourself after them -
remembering that they are not perfect -
they are on their own path toward a calm and
More positive future.

N

Nature

Nurture yourself in Nature.

Brain waves calm when we are out in Nature.

Find a park, a trail, some trees, a lake, grass, or greenspace.

Take a walk. Breathe deeply.

Notice the flowers, the greenery, the wildlife,

the bugs in the grass, the birds overhead.

Breathe deeply. Breathe again.

O

Open up
Open yourself to new experiences & friendships.
You can Overcome your past - your fears.
Open yourself to considering new activities -
Yoga, a book club, drawing, an instrument,
running, riding a bike, taking a class,
going to the gym, volunteering.
Open yourself to moving forward
in new ways.

P

Pause
Pray and/or meditate.
Know that you are not alone in the universe.
Take time to listen to that still small voice within –
breathe deeply, be still.
By Pausing, you calm yourself and open yourself to new ideas
Be Present
And set all the chaos aside.

Q

Question
Question the effects of the past on your present choices.
Query the effects of trauma.
Quiet yourself and listen for the answers -
From within, from positive people you trust,
from new experiences,
from new readings.
Engage in a Quest for new approaches to life -
moving toward a more positive future.

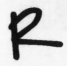

R

Reality Check

From time to time take stock.

Are you moving forward with positive choices?

Are you making progress on your goals?

Has anything or anyone deRailed you?

Do you need to Restart?

Is there additional assistance you need?

Where might you find it?

Be Real with yourself.

S

Step Programs & the Serenity Prayer

Consider a 12-Step Program.

Think about the Serenity Prayer -
taking responsibility for those things that are yours,
letting go of those things that aren't,
and having the wisdom to know the difference.

Consider AA, Alateen, Al-Anon, ACOA or other programs
to connect with others who are on a
similar journey to your own.

T

Talk

Tell your story. Tell it again.

Tell it to your confidante, mentor, counselor,

or Therapist,

your pastor, priest, rabbi, or imam.

Tell it to someone you Trust -

your support group or your best friend.

Tell it and

Tell it again until you don't need to

Tell it anymore, and its power over you is gone.

Tell your story until you are finally at peace with it.

u

understand
understand that healing takes hard work and time.
undoing the effects of trauma is tough.
Forgive yourself when you trip up and have to start
again.
undertaking healing is difficult,
but it can be done.
understand yourself and offer yourself kindness
on the journey.

V

Victories

Victories will come along the way.

Small victories - large victories.

Celebrate them all!

Celebrate anniversary dates - daily, monthly, annually.

Celebrate victories with others who are making progress on their journeys.

Mark the victories in a tangible way -

stickers in your journal; beads on your bracelet;

tally marks on your calendar.

W

Watch

Watch out for the potholes.

Watch out for the temptation to help others before you have helped yourself.

Watch out for addictions.

Watch out for guilt trips that others may try to put on you as you begin to experience success.

Be wary of negative people who would pull you from your path.

X

Exorcise and Exercise

Examine and exorcise those things that have negative effects

on you - alcohol, drugs, unstable people,

and unhealthy circumstances.

Exercise your body and your mind -

take a class; watch a Ted Talk; read; take a walk;

try bicycling or running; listen to music.

Keep your mind and body active and healthy.

Build positive addictions - to learning & bodily health!

Y

You

Focus on You!

Don't yield to the temptation to focus on others –

their chaos, their problems, their issues.

Focus on yourself and your progress.

Your hourly, daily, weekly, monthly goals.

YOu and your choices –

Your future.

Z

ZZZZZZZZZ......
Look forward to a good night's sleep –
Falling into slumber naturally at the end of a positive,
productive, and perhaps exhausting day.
Look forward to sleep without chemical assistance –
Without chaotic dreams –
Peaceful, wonderful, restful sleep.
Knowing the next day when you awaken you will be one step
further on your journey.

ABOUT THE AUTHOR

Mariah Clark Skewes is the pseudonym chosen by author Mary Boyle because of its family significance - her mum enrolled her in kindergarten under that name. As children, Mariah and her siblings considered themselves "The Three Musketeers - one for all and all for one" as they tightly bonded through the challenges of multiple childhood disruptions and displacements due to their mum's chronic schizophrenia; their father's alcoholism, abandonment, and early death; and their stepmother/guardian's alcoholism and emotional abuse. They were uniquely affected by their childhood experiences, and each chose a different path in life, but today they are happy, functional adults. Mariah/Mary holds a Bachelor's Degree in Psychology, a Master's Degree in Special Education, and multiple teaching and administrative credentials. She is the proud mother of four fabulous adult children and lives with her husband on a vineyard in Northern California where she runs daily on trails, volunteers with children in foster care, and competes in marathons around the world.

Life is not easy, nor is it fair. But it can get better.

RESOURCES

Help for Mental Illness & Crisis Line - samhsa.gov
Mental Illness Resources - nimh.nih.gov
Substance Abuse and Mental Health - samhsa.gov
Crisis Intervention - nami.org/help

JOURNAL

JOURNAL

CPSIA information can be obtained
at www.ICGtesting.com
Printed in the USA
BVHW010729090323
659963BV00008BA/383